Healthy Foods Book 2

The Ultimate Guide To Healthy Foods And Healthy Cooking!

Table Of Contents

Introduction

I know what you are thinking. It's easy for someone who has been cooking for a number of years and not only loves cooking but does it to earn a living.

Well, relax. This book is designed to help ease the burden of making the transition to a healthier, whole foods and grain foods – based diet, from introduction to grains to healthy grain recipes.

What does whole grain mean anyway? This name refers to a seed's anatomical structure- the pericarp, endosperm and germ. So, any reference to whole grains means that the entire grain structure is being used; there has been no polishing, rolling, purling or stripping of seed. All the nutritive parts of the grain are intact for consumption.

I hope these recipes will aid you on your journey towards a healthier way of eating.

Chapter 1: All About The AMAZIGN GRAINS

Grain. It's interesting how even the word evokes feelings of simplicity, elegance, beauty and humility. Simply stated, grain products and whole grains are the backbone of any healthy and also whole foods diet. There is an old saying, "Man cannot live by bread alone." But he sure can live well on grain! Yes, we need to supplement whole grains with vegetables, beans, fresh fruits and nuts, seeds, and even a small amount of fish, if you desire. Grains are the link between the plant and animal kingdoms in which we, as humans, draw life.

So are grains the whole around perfect food? Just about. The majority of nutrients that the human organism needs to sustain life are fully present in whole grains. Water, protein, vitamins, minerals , carbohydrates, fats and fiber compose this miraculous food that not only reproduces itself a thousand times over (with little assistance from us), but can be stored and transported literally without damage or spoilage.

In traditional cultures, grain was always associated with the fruitful forces of mother nature. To these people grain was the key to opening consciousness, carrying the force of life through its deep roots on earth up through its stem to its fruit, opened to the heavenly force of the sun. In modern botanical thinking, there are about eight thousand species of grasses that are categorized as "grain". Of these, human beings only eat a few, although we have come to think of other plant varieties as "grains" because of the similarities in their characteristics and energetic qualities.

When shopping for whole grains. I personally prefer organic grains to commercial varieties, because grain is such an important part of a healthy diet, it only makes sense to obtain the very best quality. And since grains absorb so much from the soil, any pesticide residue present in the earth will find its way into our grains.

Once purchased, I advise storing grains in a tightly sealed glass jar in a cupboard or pantry – or any cool dry place. I have gotten into the habit of adding a whole bay leaf to each jar to discourage grain moths. At first, with so many grains available to us, you may wish to label each jar, so you will remember what is what until grains become familiar to you.

In general, cooking styles for grains will vary – amounts of water, cooking time, etc. you will see many different methods employed in the following recipes. What remains constant is rinsing grains. Grains will develop a light dust over their surface as they sit because of their naturally occurring oxidation. A light rinsing process will ensure the natural, sweet, nutty taste of your cooked grains. First, quickly sort through the grain for any tiny stones or debris. Then, simply place the grain in a bowl, cover with water, swirl gently with your fingers to loosen dirt and pour through a fine strainer. You may wish to repeat the process a couple of times if the water is particularly cloudy.

The energy and spirit of whole grains keep me enchanted almost more than the delicious flavors. They possess an inner strength that comes from the harmony of water, earth, sun and air – nature's basic elements of life. By utilizing the whole grain, these powerful energetic qualities are passed on to us, nourishing us completely and restoring us to the same harmony with nature.

A diet centered around the grain family will awaken our spirits and open our consciousness to all that the universe has to provide. Our instinct and intuition will guide our choices, making our lives healthier and happier and free from the petty stresses of daily living that seem to so debilitate people these days.

Looking at grains, we see a great variety available to us. I dare say that, to a newcomer, a natural foods store with row after row of grain products can be quite daunting. But instead of giving in to anxiety, let this abundance reawaken the very essence of humanity in you- your creativity. And again, always choose organic grains over commercially grown and processed ones whenever possible. Organic foods nourish us better because they are allowed to flourish naturally, and they also support the earth and gives them life.

Let these recipes serve only as your inspiration. All that follows are simply tools to create dishes to nourish the body and spirit. For more information on the vast varieties of grains available to us, check on the Glossary.

Chapter 2: Grain Recipes Number 1

Mochi

made from sweet brown rice, mocha is so versatile you can use it in sauces, stews, casseroles and soups; as a cheese alternative; and on its own. While you can purchase it packaged, nothing compares to homemade mocha. Make the effort; it really is worth it.

2 cups sweet brown rice, rinsed

2 ½ cups spring or filtered water

2 pinches of sea salt

Rice flour

Place rice and water in a pressure cooker and soak 6 to 8 hours. Bring to a boil, loosely covered. Add salt, seal, and bring to full pressure. Place over a flame deflector, reduce heat to low and cook for 45 minutes. Remove pot from heat and allow pressure to reduce naturally. Transfer grain to a heavy clay or wooden bowl.

Take a large pestle and moisten it. Begin pounding the cooked rice, periodically dipping the pestle in water to prevent the rice from sticking. Continue pounding about 1 hour, until all the grains of rice appear to be broken and the rice is very sticky. Sprinkle a baking sheet with rice flour and spread mochi evenly over the sheet. Cover with a straw mat and allow to dry 1 to 2 days before cutting into pieces and wrapping in plastic. Mochi will keep, refrigerated, about 10 days. **Makes about 10 ounces**

VARIATION: Place freshly pounded mocha in a moistening plastic container. Cover and refrigerate. The mochi will be a little softer, but just as good.

Short – Grain Brown Rice with Squash

This is a staple in our house during the fall and winter, when the squash is so sweet that you'd swear it was sugared if you didn't know better. A delicious breakfast dish when cooked soft, it creates a very warming energy, which nourishes our middle body organs, like spleen, pancreas and stomach, but it will also liven up any evening meal very nicely.

2 cups short- grain brown rice, rinsed

1 cup cubed winter squash

3 cups spring or filtered water

2 pinches of sea salt

1 tablespoon barley miso

Silvered nori sheets or minced parsley, for garnish

Combine rice, squash, and water in a pressure cooker and cook over medium heat, uncovered, until mixture comes to boil. Add salt. Seal and bring to full pressure. Place over a flame deflector, reduce heat to low, and cook 50 minutes.

Meanwhile, puree miso in small amount of water and simmer it 3 to 4 minutes. When the rice is cooked, remove it from heat and allow pressure to reduce naturally. Stir pureed miso into hot rice and transfer to a serving bowl. Serve garnished with nori or parsley. **Makes 5 to 6 servings.**

Fried Rice & Vegetables

A familiar favorite. This vegetarian version relies on an abundance of fresh vegetables and flavorful seasoning to create a low- fat, delicious alternative to the oily and salty standard.

1 to 2 teaspoons dark sesame oil

3 or 4 slices gingerroot, cut into thin matchsticks

Sea salt

¼ cup each sliced onion, carrot matchsticks, burdock matchsticks, thinly sliced button mushrooms and shredded cabbage

1 to 2 cups cooked short-grain brown rice

1 to 2 stalks broccoli, broken into flowerets

Soy sauce

Brown rice vinegar

Parsley sprigs, for garnish

Heat oil in a skillet. Add gingerroot and pinch of salt and cook, stirring, until golden. Add onion and another pinch of salt and cook, stirring, until onion is translucent, about 5 minutes. Add carrot, burdock, mushrooms and another pinch of salt and cook, stirring occasionally, until coated with oil. Finally, stir in cabbage and another pinch of salt and cook until cabbage begins to wilt, about 5 minutes.

Spread vegetables evenly over the skillet and top with cooked rice, then broccoli. Sprinkle lightly with soy sauce. Gently add about 1/8 inch of water to allow everything to steam together, cover and cook over medium heat about 10 minutes, until all liquid is absorbed and broccoli is cooked. Turn off heat and season to taste with rice vinegar. Stir well, transfer to serving bowl and garnish with parsley sprigs. **Makes 4 or 5 servings**

Millet & Veggie Burgers

This is such an easy dish to put together for lunches or snacks or on those nights when you would love to just send out for pizza instead of cooking a well-balanced, healthy meal. These burgers satisfy the cook's need for ease of preparation, without compromising your food choices.

1 to 2 teaspoons light sesame oil, plus additional for pan-frying

3 to 4 slices gingerroot, cut into thin matchsticks

Sea salt

1 cup millet, rinsed

3 cups boiling water

½ cup each diced carrot, onion and celery

¼ cup minced fresh parsley

½ cup cornmeal, plus additional for dredging

Heat 1 to 2 teaspoons sesame oil in a pot of over medium heat. Add gingerroot and a pinch of salt and cook 2 to 3 minutes. Remove ginger from oil. Add millet and cook, stirring, until millet is coated with oil and gives off a nutty fragrance. Add boiling water, season lightly with salt and reduce heat to low. Cover and simmer 35 minutes. Add carrot, onion and celery, re-cover, and simmer about 5 minutes. Remove from heat and stir in parsley and cornmeal. Allow mixture to stand 10 to 15 minutes before forming into burgers.

Shape millet mixture into thick patties. Dredge in cornmeal to coat. Heat about 1/8 inch sesame oil in skillet over medium heat. Fry patties until golden, about 3 minutes on each side. Remove from skillet and drain on paper towels to absorb any excess oil. Serve as you would any conventional burger. **Makes 4 or 5 servings**

Chapter 3: Grain Recipes Number 2

Chilled Oriental Rice

It may sound like just another brown rice and tofu salad, but this delicious take on oriental traditional fare contains less salt and fat than its restaurant counterpart. It is a great easy recipe for using up leftover grain as well.

8 ounces extra-firm tofu, cubed

Marinade

7 or 8 snow peas, cut into thin slices

1 celery stalk, diced

½ red bell papper, roasted, diced

2 cups cooked medium – or long grain brown rice

2 tablespoons minced, pan- roasted walnut pieces

Sliced green onions, for garnish

MARINADE

1 to 2 teaspoons light sesame oil

Juice of 1 lemon

Juice of 1 lime

2 cloves garlic, minced

Fresh ginger juice

Soy sauce

Brown rice vinegar

Spring or filtered water

Place cubed tofu in a shallow dish. Mix together marinade ingredients, combining a little ginger juice, soy sauce and vinegar with enough water to create a thin marinade. The flavors in the marinade can be as strong or as mild as you like; because the tofu takes on the flavors of the marinade, err to the mild side on the taste here. Pour marinade over tofu and allow to stand 10 to 15 minutes.

Combine vegetables, rice, walnuts, tofu and marinade. Serve garnished with green onions. **Makes 4 or 5 servings**

Roasted Vegetable & Corn Chili

This thick, rich, elegant tasting version of a classic recipe employs corn grits as an unusual alternative to the beans usually found in vegetarian versions of chili without meat. Serve with crusty whole- grain bread and lightly boiled or steamed veggies to round out your meal.

1 to 2 yellow squash, cut into cubes

1 red bell pepper, diced

1 portobello mushrooms, cut into cubes

1 to 2 cups chopped button mushrooms

Extra-virgin olive oil

Sea salt

1 yellow onion, diced

3 cloves garlic, diced

Generous pinch each of ground cumin and powdered ginger

2 to 3 fresh plum tomatoes, diced

½ cup fresh corn kernels

Spring or filtered water

Generous pinch of chili powder

1 cup corn grits

Preheat oven to 450F (220C). Toss the squash, bell pepper and mushrooms in a little olive oil. Spread on baking sheet and sprinkle lightly with salt. Roast about 20 minutes, tossing occasionally, until lightly browned. Remove from oven and set aside.

Heat 2 teaspoons olive oil in a large, heavy Dutch oven over medium heat. Add the onion, garlic and a pinch of salt and sauté until fragrant, 2 to 3 minutes. Stir in cumin and ginger and cook 1 to 2 minutes more. Add tomatoes, corn, 3 cups water, a pinch of salt and chili powder to taste. Fold in corn grits and roasted vegetables, cover partially and simmer, stirring occasionally, over low heat until thick, about 1 hour. Add water as needed as chili cooks. The finished product should be creamy and thick, but not pasty. **Makes 4 or 5 servings**

Sweet & Sour Corn Salad

The quintessential symbol of summer, this wonderful summer grain is packed with vitamins, minerals and protein. Growing high and proud, it is at its best during the warmest summer weather. The high "fire" energy it contains gives us great vitality and helps us adapt more smoothly to the warm temperatures of the season. This salad is a different take on the use of corn: the mustard -flavored sweet and sour sauces enhances the sweet taste of the corn just perfectly. It is great served over a bed of lightly steamed leafy greens.

4 ears of fresh corn, kernels removed

1 red bell pepper, roasted over a flame, peeled, seeded and diced

½ cucumber, seeded and diced, but not peeled

3 to 4 green onions, cut into thin diagonal slices

¼ cup minced fresh parsley

SWEET & SOUR SAUCE

1 teaspoon rice syrup

½ teaspoon umeboshi vinegar

2 tablespoons spring or filtered water

Soy sauce

2 tablespoons brown rice vinegar

3 to 4 teaspoons prepared mustard

1 teaspoon extra-virgin oil

Bring a small pot of water to a boil and add the corn kernels. Return to a boil and drain. (this will enhance the sweet flavor of the corn and make it tender.) Toss together the corn, bell pepper, cucumber, onions and parsley in a large bowl.

Combine the sauce ingredients in a small bowl and whisk until blended. Stir sauce into the vegetables and allow to marinate about 30 minutes so the flavors can develop.
Makes 4 or 5 servings

Chapter 4: Grain Recipes Number 3

Rice Pilaf

No grain section would be complete without a pilaf recipe. This popular style of serving whole grains is a chewy, crunchy symphony of flavors, textures and colors.

1 teaspoon light sesame oil

1 onion, diced

Sea salt

2 tablespoons silvered almonds

1 cup thinly sliced button mushrooms, brushed clean

1 cup fresh corn kernels

1 carrot, diced

1 cup long-grain brown rice

¼ cup wild rice

2 ½ cups spring or filtered water

Parsley sprigs, for garnish

In a deep, heavy pot, heat the oil over medium heat. Add the onions and pinch of salt and cook until fragrant, 2 to 3 minutes. Add the almonds and cook, stirring, until coated with oil. Stir in the mushrooms, corn, carrot and pinch of salt and cook 1 to 2 minutes more. Spread the vegetables evenly over the bottom of the pot and top with rice (combined).

Gently add water and bring to boil. Add 1 or 2 pinches of salt. Reduce heat, cover and simmer over low heat about 45 minutes, until all the liquid is absorbed and the rices are fluffy. Remove pot from heat and allow to stand, covered, 5 minutes. Stir well and transfer to a serving bowl. Garnish with parsley sprigs. **Makes 4 or 5 servings**

Chili with Polenta Croutons

Meatless meals have predominated cooking throughout most, if not all, cultures. This peasant cuisine again becoming fashionable as modern people discover that vegetarian meals are satisfying and simple to prepare. I worked as head chef a number of years ago in natural foods restaurant where this chili recipe was developed. It is best that I have ever tasted . Its thick texture and authentic, spicy flavor will win raves. Trust me, no one will miss meat in this meal. Serve with crusty whole-grain bread and lightly cooked vegetables.

1 (1-inch) piece kombu

½ cup each pinto beans and kidney beans, soaked together 6 to 8 hours and drained

Spring or filtered water

Generous pinch of cumin powder

1 to 2 teaspoons chili powder

½ cup each diced onion, celery, winter squash and carrot

1 cup millet, rinsed

Soy sauce

About 2 teaspoons extra- virgin olive oil

1 recipe old world polenta cut into 1-inch squares

Place kombu in the bottom of a pressure cooker. Add beans and 3 cups fresh water. Bring to a boil, uncovered, over medium heat and cook at a rolling boil about 10 minutes. Seal and bring to full pressure. Reduce heat to low and cook 40 minutes. Remove pot from heat and allow pressure to reduce naturally. Open the pot, stir cumin and chili powder to taste and simmer 5 minutes, uncovered.

In a soup pot, layer the onion, celery, squash, carrot, millet and finally the cooked beans. Add water to generously cover all ingredients and sprinkle lightly with soy sauce. Cover and bring to a boil over medium heat. Reduce heat and cook 35 minutes, until millet is creamy and chili is thick and "meaty".

Heat enough olive oil in a skillet over medium heat to cover the bottom. Add polenta squares and cook, turning, until golden brown on both sides. Garnish each bowl of chili with a few polenta squares and serve. **Makes 5 or 6 servings**

VARIATION: You may also use canned organic beans instead of cooking your own to save cooking time in this recipe.

Bulgur with Skillet Veggies

 A very simple and satisfying one-dish meal. Serve with a fresh salad and a light soup to round out a refreshing summer repast.

1 to 2 teaspoons light sesame oil

1 onion, diced

1 clove garlic, minced

Sea salt

1 cup bulgur wheat

2 cups spring or filtered water

2 cups thinly sliced fresh crimini or button mushrooms brushed clean

1 cup small cauliflowerets

1 carrot, cut into thin matchsticks

7 or 8 Brussels sprouts, halved and thinly sliced lengthwise

Soy sauce

Generous pinch of dried rosemary

1 tablespoon kuzu, dissolved in a little cold water

2 tablespoons slivered almonds, pan-toasted, for garnish

Heat sesame oil in a skillet over medium heat. Add onion, garlic and a pinch of sea salt and sauté until translucent, 2 to 3 minutes. Add bulgur and cook, stirring constantly, about 2 minutes. Gently add water and a pinch of salt and bring to a boil. Cover, reduce heat, and cook 15 minutes, until liquid is absorbed.

In another skillet over medium heat, arrange mushrooms,

cauliflower, carrot and Brussels sprouts around the skillet, each in its own section. Add enough water to half cover, sprinkle lightly with soy sauce, and bring to a boil. Cover, reduce heat, and simmer until cauliflower is crisp-tender, about 6 minutes. Add rosemary to taste and stir in dissolved kuzu. Cook, stirring, until liquid is slightly thickened. Transfer bulgur to a serving bowl and top individual servings with vegetables and almonds. **Makes 4 to 5 servings**

Barley & Corn Salad

A lovely summer combination, this salad joins the cooling, dispersing energy of barley with energizing power of fresh summer corn, all generously dressed in a refreshing lime vinaigrette.

2 cups spring or filtered water

Sea salt

1 cup pearl barley, sorted and rinsed

1 to 2 ears fresh corn, kernels removed

1 small red onion, diced

1 small cucumber, peeled, seeded and diced

¼ cup minced fresh parsley

¼ cup extra-virgin olive oil

2 to 3 tablespoons umeboshi vinegar

2 teaspoons rice syrup

Juice of lime

1 to 2 tablespoons prepared mustard

Bring water and a pinch of sea salt to a boil in medium saucepan over medium heat. Slowly add barley. Cover, reduce heat to low, and cook 40 to 45 minutes, until barley is tender and water is absorbed. Transfer to a bowl and allow to cool.

Bring water to a boil in a pot over high heat. Add corn and boil 2 minutes. Remove with a slotted spoon and cool in iced water. Drain and set aside. Add onion to boiling water and boil 1 minute. Drain and cool in iced water. Drain and mix together with the corn, cucumber and parsley in a large bowl.

In a small bowl, combine the oil, umeboshi vinegar, rice syrup, lime juice, mustard and a little salt. Whisk until blended. The dressing should have a refreshing, yet spicy taste. Toss the barley, vegetables, and dressing together. Allow the salad to marinate in the refrigerator about 30 minutes before serving. **Makes 4 or 5 servings**

Chapter 5: Grain Recipes Number 5

Oriental- Style Millet

Millet is one of the wonders of the culinary world. It is one of the most versatile grains, with delicious, nutty flavor. It cooks up creamy and stew like or you can simply pan-roast it to make it fluffy and light, enhancing and supporting the other flavors in the dish, as in this elegant, exotic grain dish.

1 cup millet, rinsed

3 cups spring or filtered water

Soy sauce

1 to 2 teaspoons dark sesame oil

3 to 4 slices gingerroot, minced

2 cloves garlic, minced

1 small carrot, finely diced

2 to 3 green onions, cut into thin diagonal slices

1 teaspoon fresh ginger juice

1 teaspoon brown rice syrup

1 tablespoon brown rice vinegar

2 tablespoons shelled peanuts, pan-toasted

Heat a deep, dry skillet over medium heat. Drain millet well before toasting so that it toasts evenly and doesn't burn. Add to skillet and toast about 5 minutes, until millet puffs and begins to pop. Add water and sprinkle of soy sauce and bring to boil. Reduce heat, cover, and simmer 30 minutes or until the liquid is nearly absorbed. Remove from heat and allow to stand, covered, 10 minutes. Fluff with a fork and transfer to a serving bowl.

Heat sesame oil in a skillet over medium heat. Add ginger and garlic and cook 2 to 3 minutes. Add carrot and green onions and cook until tender, 2 to 3 minutes. Sprinkle with a little soy sauce and stir in ginger juice and rice syrup. Remove from heat and stir in rice vinegar and peanuts. Fold into hot millet. Serve warm, as millet tends to stiffen as it cools. **Makes 4 or 5 servings**

Amaranth & Corn

An ancient grain revisited. It was cultivated by the Aztecs, but was also widely used in China and South and Central America. Commonly ground into flour, amaranth is a wonderful whole-grain dish, but it only recently came back into vogue as a grain. It has a strong, earthy, sweet flavor that matches perfectly the sweetness of fresh corn. Its unique flavor and texture make it a delicious alternative to the more commonly used whole grains.

1 cup amaranth, rinsed and drained through a very fine strainer

½ cup fresh corn kernels

2 ¼ cups spring or filtered water

Pinch of sea salt

Combine amaranth, corn and water in a medium pan over medium heat and bring to a boil. Add salt. Cover, reduce heat and simmer 30 to 35 minutes, until all the liquid is absorbed and the grain is creamy. **Makes 4 or 5 servings**

VARIATION: This grain dish combines very well with hato mugi barley, also known as Job's Tears. Cooked in the same manner as the recipe indicates, you simply add ¼ cup barley to the amaranth and increase the water by a little over ½ cup.

Quinoa with Tempeh & Cilantro

Truly a fast food, quinoa cooks up very quickly, unfolding like a spiral as it cooks. As in this recipe, quinoa partners very well with more cooling vegetables and helps to create some wonderful, nutty grain dishes.

1 cup quinoa

2 cups spring or filtered water

Pinch of sea salt

Safflower oil for deep-frying

1 (8-oz.) package tempeh, cubed

1 teaspoon extra-virgin olive oil

1 clove garlic, minced

6 to 7 green onions, cut into thin diagonal slices

Soy sauce

2 celery stalks, diced

Juice of 1 lime

¼ cup cilantro, minced

Place quinoa in a fine strainer and rinse well. This is especially important because the grains are covered with a coating of a substance called saponin, which protects the delicate grains. If not rinsed off, this substance can make your cooked grain taste bitter. Place in a pot with water and bring to a boil. Add salt. Cover, reduce heat, and simmer about 30 minutes, until liquid is absorbed and quinoa is fluffy. Set aside.

Heat about 1 inch of safflower oil in a heavy skillet or pan over medium heat. Test the oil temperature by dropping in a piece of tempeh. If it sinks and comes immediately back to the top, the oil is hot enough to deep-fry properly. Deep-fry the tempeh cubes until golden brown. Drain on paper towels and set aside.

Heat olive oil in a skillet over medium heat. Add the garlic, green onions and a little soy sauce and cook until onions are bright green, about 3 minutes. Stir in celery, quinoa, and tempeh and toss well. Remove from heat and stir in lime juice and cilantro. Serve warm. **Makes 4 or 5 servings**

Brown Rice & Millet Croquettes

Tired of simply re-steaming leftover grain, putting it into soup or , even worse, throwing it away after a few days? Well, this recipe is for you. All you need to make croquettes is some cooked grains, some oil and about half an hour to prepare the dish. The amounts suggested are really just a guide. Grain ratios may vary, depending on what you have available. The same goes for vegetables.

½ cup cooked brown rice

½ cup cooked millet

¼ cup combined diced onion and carrot

¼ cup fresh corn kernels (optional)

Fine yellow or white cornmeal

Safflower oil for deep-frying or shallow frying

Combine grains and vegetables in a large bowl. With moist hands, form the croquettes into small rounds, thick discs or oblong fingers. Pour some cornmeal onto a plate and gently pat croquette until completely coated. This will hold the croquette together as well as give its crispy outer coating.

To deep- fry, heat about 1 inch of oil in a heavy skillet or pan over medium heat. Deep-fry each croquette until golden brown. Drain well on paper towels to remove excess oil. If shallow-frying, heat about ¼ inch of oil in a skillet over medium heat. Fry the croquettes on each side until golden brown. Drain well on paper towels.

These are great served with creamy sesame dressing, garlic, mushroom & leek sauce or a simple dipping sauce consisting of soy sauce, water and fresh ginger juice or lemon juice.
Makes 4 or 5 servings

VARIATIONS: Don't be limited to this combination. Any cooked whole or cracked grains will make delicious croquettes. Rice with bulgur, millet with couscous, barley and corn- the list is virtually endless.

Bulgur, Mushroom & Greens Salad

In the summer months, it is really nice to lighten things up a bit with quick- cooking cracked grains on occasion. This delicious salad combines a variety of flavors to create a nutty, sweet and sour medley.

2 cups spring or filtered water

Sea salt

1 cup bulgur

2 tablespoons extra-virgin olive oil

½ cup diced onion

1 cup button mushrooms, brushed clean and thinly sliced

6 or 7 leaves kale or collard greens, rinsed

1 cup seedless grapes

Juice of one lemon

2 tablespoons slivered almonds, pan- toasted

Bring water and a pinch of salt to a boil in medium pan over medium heat. Add bulgur, cover, and reduce heat. Cook 20 minutes or until water is absorbed and bulgur is fluffy.

Heat oil in a skillet over medium heat. Add onion and a pinch of salt and cook until translucent, about 5 minutes. Add mushrooms and sauté until limp. Slice greens into small pieces, add to the skillet and cook 10 minutes or until greens are deep green. Add grapes and stir well. Remove from heat and stir in lemon juice. Toss with bulgur and almonds and transfer to serving bowl. **Makes 4 or 5 servings**

NOTE: Pan-toast almonds in a dry skillet over medium heat, stirring constantly, until fragrant, about 5 minutes.

Conclusion

Thank you for purchasing this book on *Healthy Foods And Cooking*....

I am extremely excited to pass this information along to you, and I am so happy that you now have read and can hopefully implement these strategies going forward.

I hope this book was able to help you understand the basic idea of eating well and how to shop for healthy foods.

The next step is to get started using this information and to hopefully live a healthier yet frugal life! Please don't be someone who just reads this information and doesn't apply it, the strategies in this book will only benefit you if you use them!

If you know of anyone else that could benefit from the information presented here please inform them of this book.

Finally, if you enjoyed this book and feel it has added value to your life in any way, please take the time to share your thoughts and post a review on Amazon. It'd be greatly appreciated!

Thank you and good luck!

Legal Notice

Disclaimer Notice

omissions, or inaccuracies. Because of the rate with which conditions change, the author and publisher reserve the right to alter and update the information contained herein on the new conditions whenever they see applicable.